TABLE OF CONTENT

INTRODUCTION

Welcome to the Total Manual for Labrador Retrievers! Whether you're a first-time Labrador proprietor or a carefully prepared reproducer, this far reaching manual is intended to give you all the data you really want to comprehend, care for, and partake in these magnificent canines. Labrador Retrievers, frequently basically called "Labs," are one of the most famous canine varieties on the planet, and for good explanation. With their agreeable attitude, knowledge, and flexibility,

Labs make brilliant family pets, administration canines, treatment canines, and working canines in different fields like pursuit and salvage, hunting, and location.

In this manual, we'll begin by diving into the captivating history and beginning of the Labrador Retriever breed. From their modest starting points as fishing and hunting friends in Newfoundland to their ascent as darling family pets across the globe, you'll figure out how Labs have caught the hearts of millions.

The Labrador Retriever or essentially Labrador is an English variety of retriever firearm canine. It was created in the Unified Realm from St. John's water canines imported from the state of Newfoundland (presently a territory of Canada), and was named after the Labrador district of that settlement. It is among the most normally kept canines in a few nations, especially in the European world.

The Labrador is agreeable, lively, and fun loving. It was reproduced as a brandishing and hunting canine yet is broadly kept as a buddy canine. It might likewise be prepared as an aide or help canine, or for salvage or treatment work.

During the 1830s, the tenth Baron of Home and his nephews, the fifth Duke of Buccleuch and Ruler John Scott, imported ancestors of the variety from Newfoundland to Europe for use as weapon canines. One more early supporter of these Newfoundland fishing canines was the second Baron of Malmesbury, who reproduced them for their aptitude in waterfowling.

During the 1880s, the third Lord of Malmesbury, the sixth Duke of Buccleuch, and the twelfth Baron of Home teamed up to create and lay out the Labrador Retriever breed. The canines Buccleuch Avon and Buccleuch Ned, given by Malmesbury to Buccleuch, were mated with bitches conveying blood from those initially imported by the fifth Duke and the tenth Lord of Home. The posterity are the precursors of every cutting edge Labrador.

LABRADOR RETRIEVER HISTORY

Labrador Retrievers hail from the island of Newfoundland, off the northeastern Atlantic shoreline of Canada. Initially called St. John's canines, after the capital city of Newfoundland, Labs filled in as sidekicks and partners to the nearby anglers starting during the 1700s. The canines went through their days working close by their proprietors, recovering fish who had gotten away from snares and towing in lines, and afterward got back to go through the night with the anglers' loved ones.

Despite the fact that their legacy is obscure, many trust the St. John's canine was interbred with the Newfoundland Canine and other little neighborhood water canines. Pariahs saw the canine's handiness and great demeanor, and English athletes imported a couple of Labs to Britain to act as retrievers for hunting. The second Duke of Malmesbury was quite possibly the earliest, and had St. John's canines transported to Britain at some point around 1830.

The third Lord of Malmesbury was the primary individual to allude to the canines as Labradors. Incredibly, Labs-now America's most famous canine were practically terminated by the 1880s, and the Malmesbury family and other English fans are credited with saving the variety. In Newfoundland, the variety vanished in light of government limitations and assessment regulations. Families were permitted to keep something like one canine, and claiming a female was exceptionally burdened, so young lady doggies were separated from litters.

In Britain, notwithstanding, the variety made due, and the Pet hotel Club perceived the Labrador Retriever as a particular variety in 1903. The American Pet hotel Club stuck to this same pattern in 1917, and during the '20s and '30s, English Labs were imported to lay out the variety in the U.S. The variety's notoriety truly started to take off after The Second Great War, and in 1991, the Labrador Retriever turned into the most famous canine enlisted with the American Pet hotel Club-and they've held that differentiation from that point onward. They likewise top the rundown in Canada and Britain. Today, Labs work in medication and unstable location, search and salvage, treatment, help to those with handicaps, and as retrievers for trackers. They additionally succeed in all types of canine contests: show, field, spryness, and submission.

LABRADOR RETRIEVER SIZES

Males stand 22.5 to 24.5 inches, and weigh 65 to 80 pounds. Females stand 21.5 to 23.5 inches, and weigh 55 to 70 pounds.

BEFORE BREEDING: PREPARATIONS AND ARRANGEMENT

Breeding a Labrador Retrievers is a critical obligation that requires cautious preparation, information, and devotion to guarantee the wellbeing and government assistance of both the parent canines and their posterity. In this segment, we'll investigate the fundamental stages to take before setting out on the reproducing venture. Before you venture into reproducing you must take note of the three points listed below:

(1)Significance of Dependable breeding Practices

Capable breeding practices are foremost to keeping up with the wellbeing, disposition, and generally prosperity of the Labrador Retriever breed. Breeding ought to never be embraced gently or for simply monetary profit. All things considered, dependable reproducers focus on the improvement of the variety and stick to moral guidelines that focus on the wellbeing and government assistance of the canines.

(2)Choosing Reasonable Rearing Matches

Picking the right rearing pair is a basic choice that establishes the groundwork for the future wellbeing and personality of the doggies. While choosing rearing canines, it's fundamental to consider factors, for example, wellbeing, disposition, adaptation to raise guidelines, and hereditary variety. Capable raisers direct careful examination and wellbeing screenings to guarantee that both the sire and dam are liberated from inherited medical problems that could be given to their posterity.

(3)Making a Reproducing Plan

When reasonable reproducing matches have been chosen and wellbeing really looks at finished, now is the right time to make a rearing arrangement. This plan ought to frame key subtleties like the planning of reproducing, the strategy for rearing (regular mating or managed impregnation), and alternate courses of action in the event of entanglements during pregnancy or whelping.

PRE-BREEDING WELLBEING CHECKS AND HEREDITARY TESTING

Before breeding, both the male and female Labrador Retrievers ought to go through extensive wellbeing checks and hereditary testing to recognize any potential wellbeing worries that could influence the litter. Normal wellbeing screenings for Labs might incorporate hip and elbow dysplasia assessments, ophthalmic tests, and hereditary testing for genetic circumstances like moderate retinal decay (PRA) and work out actuated breakdown (EIC). By directing pre-breeding wellbeing checks and hereditary testing, reproducers can pursue informed choices to limit the gamble of genetic medical problems in the pups and guarantee that both parent canines are in ideal wellbeing for reproducing.

LABRADOR RETRIEVER PERSONALITY

The Lab has the standing of being one of the most sweet-natured breeds, and it's merited. They're cordial, anxious to please, and agreeable with the two individuals and different creatures. Beside a triumphant character, they have the insight and energy to satisfy that make them simple to prepare.

Preparing is most certainly essential since this breed has a ton of energy and extravagance. The functioning legacy of the Lab implies they are dynamic. This breed needs action, both physical and mental, to keep them cheerful. There is some variety in the action level of Labs: some are boisterous, others are more easygoing. All blossom with movement.

LABRADOR RETRIEVER HEALTH

Labrador Retrievers are by and large sound, however like all varieties, they're inclined to specific medical issue. Not all Labs will get any or these illnesses, however it's critical to know about them on the off chance that you're thinking about this variety.

(1) Hip Dysplasia: Hip dyplasia is a heritable condition wherein the thighbone doesn't fit cozily into the hip joint. A few canines show torment and weakness on one or both back legs, however you may

not see any indications of distress in a canine with hip dysplasia. As the canine ages, joint pain can create. X-beam evaluating for hip dysplasia is finished by the Muscular Starting point for Creatures or the College of Pennsylvania Hip Improvement Program. Canines with hip dysplasia ought not be reproduced.

(2)Elbow Dysplasia: This is a heritable condition normal to enormous variety canines. It's believed to be brought about by various development paces of the three bones that make up the canine's elbow, causing joint laxity. This can prompt difficult faltering. Your vet might prescribe a medical procedure to address the issue or prescription to control the aggravation.

(3)Osteochondrosis Dissecans (OCD): This muscular condition, brought about by ill-advised development of ligament in the joints, normally happens in the elbows, yet it has been found in the shoulders, also. It influences an excruciating solidifying of the joint, to the point that the canine can't twist his elbow. It tends to be distinguished in canines as soon as four to nine months old enough. Overloading of "development recipe" doggy food varieties or high-protein food varieties might add to its turn of events.

(4)Waterfalls: As in people, canine waterfalls are portrayed by shady spots on the eye focal point that can develop after some time. They might create at whatever stage in life, and frequently don't debilitate vision, albeit a few cases cause serious vision misfortune. Reproducing canines ought to be inspected by a board-guaranteed veterinary ophthamologist to be ensured as liberated from genetic eye sickness before they're reared. Waterfalls can as a rule be precisely eliminated with great outcomes.

(5)Moderate Retinal Decay (PRA): PRA is a group of eye illnesses that includes the continuous disintegration of the retina. From the get-go in the sickness, canines become night-blind. As the sickness advances, they lose their daytime vision, too. Many canines adjust to restricted or complete vision misfortune quite well, as long as their environmental elements continue as before.

(6)Epilepsy: Labs can experience the ill effects of epilepsy, which causes gentle or serious seizures. Seizures might be shown by strange way of behaving, for example, running madly as though being pursued, faltering, or stowing away. Seizures are alarming to watch, yet the drawn out visualization for canines with idiopathic epilepsy is for the most part awesome. It's memorable's vital that seizures can be brought about by numerous different things than idiopathic epilepsy, like metabolic problems, irresistible illnesses that influence the mind, growths, openness to harms, extreme head wounds, from there, the sky is the limit. In this manner, in the event that your Lab has seizures, it's critical to take them to the vet immediately for an exam.

(7)Tricuspid Valve Dysplasia (TVD): TVD is an intrinsic heart imperfection that has been expanding in pervasiveness in the Labrador breed. Little dogs are brought into the world with TVD, which is a contortion of the tricuspid valve on the right half of the heart. It tends to be gentle or serious; a few canines live without any side effects, others pass on. TVD is recognized by ultrasound. Research is continuous to figure out how boundless it is in the variety, as well as treatment.

(8)Myopathy: Myopathy influences the muscles and sensory system. The main signs are seen right on time, as youthful as about a month and a half and frequently by seven months old enough. A doggy with myopathy is drained, firm when he strolls and runs. He might fall after work out. In time, the muscles decay and the canine can scarcely stand or walk. There is no treatment, yet rest and keeping the canine warm appears to diminish side effects. Canines with myopathy ought not be reared in light of the fact that it is viewed as a heritable sickness.

(9)Gastric Dilataion-Volvulus: Regularly called swell, this is a dangerous condition that influences huge, profound chested canines like Labs, particularly assuming that they're taken care of one enormous feast a day, eat quickly, or hydrate or exercise vivaciously in the wake of eating. Bulge happens when the stomach is stretched with gas or air and afterward bends. The canine can't burp or regurgitation to free themselves of the overabundance air in their stomach, and blood stream to the heart is hindered. Circulatory strain drops and the canine goes into shock. Without quick clinical consideration, the canine can kick the bucket. Suspect bulge in the event that your canine has an enlarged mid-region, is slobbering unnecessarily, and regurgitating without hurling.

Theyalso might be fretful, discouraged, lazy, and powerless with a fast pulse. In the event that you notice these side effects, get your canine to the vet straightaway.

(10)Intense Soggy Dermatitis: Intense sodden dermatitis is a skin condition in which the skin red and kindled. It is brought about by a bacterial contamination. The more normal name of this wellbeing concern is problem areas. Treatment incorporates cutting the hair, washing in sedated cleanser, and anti-toxins.

(11)Cold Tail: Cold tail is a harmless, however difficult condition normal to Labs and different retrievers. Additionally caused agile tail, it made the canine's tail go limp. The canine might chomp at the tail. It isn't reason to worry, and generally disappears on its own in a couple of days. Being an issue with the muscles between the vertebrae in the tail is thought.

(12)Ear Contaminations: The Lab's adoration for water, joined with their drop ear make them inclined to ear diseases. Week after week checking and cleaning in the event that vital forestalls contamination.

LABRADOR RETRIEVER CARE

The adorable Lab should be around their family, and is most certainly not a patio canine. In the event that they're abandoned for a really long time, they'll most likely stain their pious standing: A desolate, exhausted Lab is well-suited to dig, bite, or track down other damaging source for their energy. Labs show some variety in their action levels, yet every one of them need movement, both physical and mental. Everyday 30-minute strolls, a cavort at the canine park, or a round of get, are a couple of ways of assisting your Lab with consuming off energy. Be that as it may, a doggy ought not be gone for a really long time strolls and ought to play for a couple of moments all at once. Labrador Retrievers are thought of "obsessive workers," and will deplete themselves. It ultimately depends on you to end play and instructional courses. Labs have such great notorieties that a few proprietors figure they don't require preparing. That is a serious mix-up. Without preparing, a raucous Lab pup will before long develop to be an exceptionally enormous, boisterous canine.

Fortunately, Labs take to preparing great; as a matter of fact, they frequently succeed in submission contests. Begin with little dog kindergarten, which shows your little guy great canine habits, yet assists them with figuring out how to be agreeable around different canines and individuals. Search for a class that involves positive preparation strategies that reward the canine for taking care of business, instead of rebuffing them for missing the point entirely. You'll have to take unique consideration on the off chance that you're raising a Lab little dog.

Try not to let your Lab little dog run and play on extremely hard surfaces, for example, asphalt until they're something like two years of age and their joints are full grown. Typical play on grass is fine, as is doggy dexterity, with its one-inch bounces. Like all retrievers, the Lab is loud, and they're most joyful when they have something, anything, to convey in their mouth. They're likewise a chewer, so make certain to keep strong toys accessible all the time-except if you need your lounge chair bit up. What's more, when you take off from the house, it's wise to keep your Lab in a container or pet hotel so they can't find themselves mixed up with inconvenience biting things they shouldn't take note.

LABRADOR'S PREGNANCY AND WHELPING PROCESS

Welcoming a litter of Labrador Retriever's pups into the world is a thrilling and compensating experience, yet it likewise requires cautious preparation and readiness to guarantee the wellbeing and prosperity of the hopeful mother and her little dogs. In this segment, we'll investigate what's in store during pregnancy and whelping and give significant direction on the most proficient method to really focus on the pregnant bitch and her infant pups.

During pregnancy, otherwise called incubation, it's vital to give the pregnant bitch appropriate consideration and nourishment to help her wellbeing and the advancement of her little dogs. Here are a few fundamental ways to really focus on a pregnant Labrador's:

(1)Nourishment: Feed a top notch, adjusted diet formed for pregnant and nursing canines. Guarantee the eating routine is wealthy in fundamental supplements like protein, calcium, and folic corrosive to help fetal turn of events.

(2)Work out: Keep on giving standard, moderate activity for the pregnant bitch to keep up with her muscle tone and generally speaking wellbeing. Stay away from demanding exercises or extreme activity that could cause injury or stress.

(3)Veterinary Consideration: Timetable normal veterinary check-ups all through the pregnancy to screen the bitch's wellbeing and the advancement of the pregnancy. Examine inoculation plans, parasite anticipation, and some other wellbeing worries with your veterinarian.

(4)Solace: Give an agreeable and calm settling region for the pregnant bitch to rest and plan for whelping. Consider utilizing a whelping box fixed with delicate sheet material to give a free from even a hint of harm climate for the birthing system.

SIGNS OF LABOR AND WHELPING

As the pregnancy advances,you should be at alert at all times,it's fundamental to find out about the indications of work and be ready for the whelping system. Signs that the bitch is approaching work might include:

(1)Anxiety

(2)Settling conduct

(3)Decrease in internal heat level

(4)Loss of craving

(5)Stomach withdrawals

When work starts, it's vital for screen the bitch intently and give help if necessary. The whelping system ordinarily happens in three phases: stage one (pre-work), stage two (dynamic work and conveyance), and stage three (ejection of the placenta).

Helping During Whelping:

While Labrador Retrievers are by and large great moms and fit for whelping and really focusing on their young doggies without help, it's fundamental to be ready to mediate in the event that entanglements emerge. Normal issues during whelping may incorporate delayed work, dystocia (trouble conceiving an offspring), and fetal misery.

Assuming you suspect that the labrador is encountering confusions during whelping, contact your veterinarian promptly for direction and help.

NEWBORN PUPPY CARE

Caring for newborn Labrador Retriever puppies during the neonatal period is a critical responsibility that requires attention to detail and a nurturing touch. In this section, we'll explore the essentials of newborn puppy care, including nutrition, temperature regulation, and early socialization.

Neonatal Care and Handling:

The neonatal period, which spans from birth to around two weeks of age, is a crucial time for the development and growth of

Labrador Retriever puppies. During this period, puppies are entirely dependent on their mother and require round-the-clock care and attention. During the neonatal period, proper nutrition is essential for supporting the growth and development of Labrador Retriever puppies. Here are some guidelines for feeding and nutrition:

(1)Colostrum: Ensure that each puppy receives adequate colostrum from the mother in the first 24 hours of life to receive essential antibodies and nutrients.

Nursing: Monitor the puppies' nursing behavior and ensure that each puppy is receiving sufficient milk from the mother. If necessary, supplement nursing with bottle feeding using a commercial canine milk replacer.

(2)Feeding Schedule: Newborn puppies typically nurse every 1-2 hours, including overnight. Establish a feeding schedule that ensures each puppy receives frequent nourishment and monitor their weight gain to ensure adequate growth.

Here are some essential aspects of newborn puppy care:

(1)Temperature Regulation: Newborn puppies are unable to regulate their body temperature effectively and rely on external sources of warmth to stay comfortable. Ensure that the whelping area is kept warm and draft-free, and consider using a heat lamp or heating pad to provide supplemental heat if necessary.

(2)Feeding and Nutrition: In the first few days of life, newborn puppies rely on colostrum, the nutrient-rich milk produced by the mother, to receive essential antibodies and nutrients. As the puppies grow, they will transition to nursing from the mother's milk. Monitor the puppies' weight gain and ensure that each puppy is nursing effectively.

(3)Stimulation and Elimination: Newborn puppies require assistance with urination and defecation until they are capable of eliminating on their own. After each feeding, use a warm, damp cloth to gently massage the puppies' genital area to stimulate elimination.

(4)Monitoring Health: Keep a close eye on the health and well-being of the newborn puppies, including monitoring for signs of distress, lethargy, or failure to thrive. Contact your veterinarian if you have any concerns about the health of the puppies.

EARLY SOCIALIZATION AND STIMULATION

Early socialization and stimulation are crucial for helping Labrador Retriever puppies develop into well-adjusted and confident adult dogs. While the neonatal period is primarily focused on basic care and nutrition, it's never too early to begin gentle handling and positive interactions with the puppies.

Handle the puppies gently and frequently to accustom them to human touch and help them become comfortable with handling as they grow. Provide opportunities for gentle play and interaction with littermates to promote socialization and development.

LABRADOR RETRIEVER FEEDING

Recommended daily amount: 2.5 to 3 cups of high-quality dry food a day, divided into two meals.

Note: How much your adult dog eats depends on their size, age, build, metabolism, and activity level. Dogs are individuals, just like people, and they don't all need the same amount of food. It almost goes without saying that a highly active dog will need more than a couch potato dog. The quality of dog food you buy also makes a difference—the better the dog food, the further it will go toward nourishing your dog and the less of it you'll need to shake into your dog's bowl.

Keep your Lab in good shape by measuring their food and feeding them twice a day rather than leaving food out all the time. If you're unsure whether they're overweight, give them the eye test and the hands-on test. First, look down at them. You should be able to see a waist. Then place your hands on their back, thumbs along the spine, with the fingers spread downward. You should be able to feel but not see their ribs without having to press hard. If you can't, they need less food and more exercise.

You'll need to take special care if you're raising a Lab puppy. These dogs grow very rapidly between the age of four and seven months, making them susceptible to bone disorders. Feed your puppy a high-quality, low-calorie diet that keeps them from growing too fast.

NUTRITION AND EXERCISE

Giving legitimate nourishment and customary activity are fundamental parts of raising a solid and cheerful Labrador Retriever dog. In this part, we'll investigate the significance of sustenance and exercise for dogs and give viable tips to guaranteeing they get a fair eating regimen and satisfactory actual work.

Nutrition for Labrador Retriever Puppies: Sustenance assumes a pivotal part in the development and improvement of Labrador Retriever young doggies. A decent eating routine that meets their particular dietary necessities is fundamental for advancing ideal wellbeing and prosperity. Here are a few vital contemplations for taking care of your Labrador Retriever pup:

(1)Pup Food: Pick a great little dog food that is explicitly figured out to meet the wholesome necessities of developing pups. Search for food sources named as "complete and adjusted" by the Relationship of American Feed Control Authorities (AAFCO).

(2)Taking care of Timetable: Lay out a customary taking care of timetable with different little feasts over the course of the day to oblige your pup's quick digestion and forestall gorging. Most pups blossom with three to four feasts each day until they are around a half year old.

(3)Segment Control: Try not to overload your pup, as abundance weight gain can prompt medical conditions sometime down the road. Adhere to the taking care of rules given by the maker in view of your little dog's age, weight, and action level.

(4)Hydration: Guarantee that your pup approaches new, clean water consistently to forestall parchedness and backing appropriate absorption and in general wellbeing.

EXERCISE AND PHYSICAL ACTIVITY

Labrador Retrievers are vivacious and athletic canines that require standard activity to keep up with their physical and mental prosperity. Here are a few ways to give satisfactory activity to your Labrador Retriever dog:

(1)Day to day Strolls: Take your little dog for day to day strolls to give mental excitement and actual activity. Begin with short strolls and step by step increment the term and power as your little dog develops.

(2)Recess: Draw in your little dog in intuitive play meetings with toys like balls, frisbees, and pull ropes. Recess gives practice as well as reinforces the connection among you and your pup.

(3)Swimming: Numerous Labrador Retrievers love to swim, on account of their water-safe coat and normal ability to swim. In the event that you approach a protected swimming region, like a pool or lake, consider acquainting your pup with water and empowering swimming as a type of activity.

(4)Preparing Exercises: Integrate preparing activities, for example, compliance preparing, nimbleness courses, and recovering games into your pup's everyday daily practice. Preparing exercises give actual activity as well as mental excitement and potential open doors for holding.

LABRADOR RETRIEVER HEALTH AND VETERINARY CARE

Guaranteeing the wellbeing and prosperity of Labrador Retriever young doggies requires proactive veterinary consideration and regard for their novel wellbeing needs. In this part, we'll investigate the significance of medical services for doggies, including immunization plans, parasite counteraction, and routine veterinary check-ups.

Inoculation Timetables

Inoculations are fundamental for safeguarding Labrador Retriever little dogs from possibly lethal irresistible sicknesses. Here are a few key inoculations that little dogs ought to get:

(1)Center Immunizations: Center antibodies safeguard against infections that are far and wide and exceptionally infectious. Center immunizations for pups ordinarily incorporate antibodies for sickness, parvovirus, adenovirus (hepatitis), and rabies.

(2)Non-Center Immunizations: Non-center antibodies might be suggested in light of the little dog's way of life and hazard of openness to explicit illnesses. Instances of non-center immunizations incorporate antibodies for leptospirosis, Bordetella (pet hotel hack), and Lyme sickness.

It's vital to follow your veterinarian's prescribed immunization timetable to guarantee that your little dog gets opportune security against preventable infections because they the once that will examine you dog.

Parasite Avoidance

Parasites represent a huge danger to the strength of Labrador Retriever little dogs and can cause a scope of issues, including digestive parasites, bugs, ticks, and heartworm sickness. Here are some fundamental parasite counteraction measures:

(1)Deworming: Young doggies ought to be regularly dewormed to dispose of normal gastrointestinal parasites like roundworms, hookworms, and whipworms. Deworming prescription is ordinarily regulated at normal spans beginning since early on.

(2)Insect and Tick Control: Utilize veterinary-supported bug and tick safeguards to shield your pup from pervasions and tick-borne illnesses like Lyme infection and ehrlichiosis. Normal preparing and examination for bugs and ticks are likewise significant.

(3)Heartworm Counteraction: Heartworm infection is a serious and possibly deadly condition sent by mosquitoes. Direct month to month heartworm safeguards as prescribed by your veterinarian to shield your doggy from this lethal parasite.

Routine Veterinary Check-ups

Standard veterinary check-ups are fundamental for observing your Labrador Retriever doggy's wellbeing and identifying any potential issues early. During veterinary arrangements, your veterinarian will lead an intensive actual assessment, regulate inoculations, examine parasite counteraction, and address any various forms of feedback you might have.

Crisis Readiness

It's critical to be ready for crises and understand what to do in the event that your pup encounters an unexpected sickness or injury. Keep a rundown of crisis contact numbers, including your veterinarian and the closest crisis veterinary facility, and really get to know normal indications of disease in doggies, like dormancy, regurgitating, loose bowels, and trouble relaxing.

By focusing on wellbeing and veterinary consideration for your Labrador Retriever little dog, you can assist with guaranteeing a long period of bliss and prosperity for your shaggy friend.

LABRADOR RETRIEVER COAT COLORS AND GROOMING

The smooth and simple consideration Sterile garment has two layers: a short, thick, straight topcoat, and a delicate, climate safe undercoat. The two-layer coat safeguards them from the cold and wet, which helps them in their job as a retriever for trackers. The coat comes in three tones: chocolate, dark, and yellow. Dark was the most loved variety among early reproducers, however throughout the long term, yellow and chocolate Labs have become well known.

A few raisers have as of late started selling "uncommon" hued Labrador Retrievers, like polar white or fox red. These shades aren't exactly interesting they're a variety of the yellow Lab. Prepping doesn't get a lot more straightforward than with a Lab, yet the variety sheds — a great deal. Purchase a quality vacuum cleaner and brush your canine everyday, particularly while they're shedding, to get out the free hair. Labs need a shower about at regular intervals or so to keep them looking perfect and smelling wonderful.bvObviously, in the event that your Lab rolls in a mud puddle or something foul, which they're able to do, it's fine to wash them on a more regular basis. Clean your Lab's teeth something like a few times each week to eliminate tartar development and the microscopic organisms that prowl inside it. Everyday brushing is far better to forestall gum illness and terrible breath. Trim nails on more than one occasion per month on the off chance that your canine doesn't wear them out normally. In the event that you can hear them tapping on the floor, they're excessively lengthy. Short, perfectly managed nails keep the feet looking great and keep your legs from getting scratched when your Lab energetically bounces up to welcome you.

Their ears ought to be checked week by week for redness or a terrible scent, which can show a contamination. At the point when you really take a look at your canine's ears, clear them out with a cotton ball hosed with delicate, pH-adjusted ear cleaner to assist with forestalling diseases. Embed nothing into the ear channel; simply clean the external ear. Since ear diseases are normal in Labs, likewise wipe out the ears after washing, swimming, or any time your canine gets wet.

Start acclimating your Lab to being brushed and inspected when they're a pup. Handle their paws regularly canines are delicate about their feet-and look inside their mouth. Make preparing a positive encounter loaded up with commendation and rewards, and you'll lay the basis for simple veterinary tests and other taking care of when they're a grown-up. As you groom, check for wounds, rashes, or indications of disease like redness, delicacy, or irritation on the skin, in the nose, mouth, and eyes, and on the feet. It would be ideal for eyes to be clear, with no redness or release. Your cautious week by week test will assist you with spotting potential medical issues early.

LABRADOR RETRIEVER CHILDREN AND OTHER PETS

The Labrador Retriever not just loves kids, they partake in the upheaval they carry with them. They'll cheerfully go to a kid's birthday celebration, and even energetically wear a party cap. Like all canines, be that as it may, they should be prepared acceptable behavior around endlessly kids should be shown acceptable behavior around the canine.

Likewise with each variety, you ought to constantly show kids how to approach and contact canines, and consistently direct any connections among canines and small kids to forestall any gnawing or ear or tail pulling with respect to one or the other party.

Show your youngster never to move toward any canine while they're eating or resting or to attempt to remove the canine's food. No canine, regardless of how cordial, ought to at any point be left solo with a youngster. On the off chance that a Lab has had a lot of openness to different canines, felines, and little creatures, and has been prepared how to communicate with them, they'll be cordial with different pets, as well.

HOW TO BUILD A STRONG BOND WITH YOUR LABRADOR

Building areas of strength for a with your Labrador is fundamental for a satisfying and amicable relationship. Labradors are known for their devotion and tender nature, and cultivating a profound association with your shaggy companion can improve both your lives. Here are a few hints on the most proficient method to reinforce the bond with your Labrador:

(1)Quality Time Together: Invest quality energy with your Labrador consistently. Whether it's taking strolls, playing bring in the lawn, or essentially nestling on the love seat, normal connection helps assemble trust and fortifies your bond.

(2)Preparing and Encouraging feedback: Take part in encouraging feedback instructional courses with your Labrador. Showing new orders and deceives invigorates your canine's brain as well as extends the connection between you as you cooperate collectively. Use rewards like treats, acclaim, and toys to support wanted ways of behaving.

(3)Actual Warmth: Show your Labrador actual warmth through delicate petting, tummy rubs, and embraces. Actual touch is a significant way for canines to feel adored and associated with their proprietors. Get some margin to scratch behind their ears or give them a back rub, building up your bond through touch.

(4)Figuring out Your Labrador's Requirements:Focus on your Labrador's signals and non-verbal communication to more readily grasp their requirements and feelings. Perceiving when they're cheerful, restless, or needing solace assists you with answering fittingly, fortifying the trust between you.

(5)Consistency and Schedule: Laying out a steady normal gives your Labrador a conviction that all is good and consistency, which can fortify your bond. Stick to standard taking care of times, work-out schedules, and sleep time ceremonies to establish a steady climate for your canine.

(6)Investigating New Undertakings Together:Take your Labrador on new undertakings and encounters to make shared recollections. Whether it's climbing in the mountains, visiting the ocean side, or investigating another canine park, encountering new conditions together fortifies your bond and builds up your association.

(7)Viable Correspondence: Openness is absolutely vital for any relationship, including the one you have with your Labrador. Utilize clear and reliable prompts to convey your assumptions and wants. Figure out how to grasp your canine's vocalizations, non-verbal communication, and looks to impart all the more successfully.

(8)Recess and Intelligent Games: Integrate recess and intelligent games into your everyday daily practice. Labradors are fun loving commonly and appreciate games like get, back-and-forth, and find the stowaway. These exercises give actual activity as well as reinforce the connection among you and your canine through shared tomfoolery and chuckling.

(9)Persistence and Understanding: Building areas of strength for a takes time, persistence, and understanding. Show restraint toward your Labrador as they learn and develop, and consistently approach cooperations with benevolence and compassion. Commend progress and victories, regardless of how little, and pardon botches en route.

(10)Unrestricted Love and Acknowledgment: Most importantly, show your Labrador unqualified love and acknowledgment. Acknowledge them for what their identity is, characteristics and all, and appreciate the interesting bond you share. Your Labrador will respond this affection and commitment, making a bond that endures forever.

LABRADOR RETRIEVER BREED ORGANIZATIONS

Finding a respectable canine reproducer is perhaps of the main choice you will make while bringing another canine into your life. Trustworthy raisers are focused on reproducing sound, all around mingled pups that will make extraordinary mates. They will evaluate their reproducing stock for medical issues, associate their little dogs since early on, and give you lifetime support. Then again, lawn reproducers are more keen on creating a gain than in delivering sound, balanced canines.

They may not evaluate their reproducing stock for medical issues, and they may not associate their pups appropriately. Therefore, little dogs from patio reproducers are bound to have both wellbeing and social issues."Taking everything into account, Labrador Retrievers are something beyond pets; they're esteemed individuals from our families, steadfast sidekicks, and wellsprings of interminable delight. All through this aide, we've investigated the fundamental components of really focusing on and holding with these brilliant canines.

CONCLUSION

As we've taken in the significance of value time spent together, the force of encouraging feedback preparing, and the meaning of grasping our Labrador's necessities and ways of behaving. We've examined the job of consistency, persistence, and sympathy in cultivating areas of strength for a, and we've praised the extraordinary association that structures between Labrador proprietors and their fuzzy companions.

As you set out on your excursion with your Labrador, recollect that building serious areas of strength for an is a continuous interaction — one that requires commitment, persistence, and love. Love every second spent together, embrace the extraordinary character of your Labrador, and proceed to learn and become together.

I need to stretch out my sincerest appreciation to you for getting some margin to peruse this aide and for your obligation to giving the most ideal consideration to your Labrador sidekick. Keep in mind, you're in good company in this excursion. There are assets accessible, networks to associate with, and experts to help you en route.

Thus, here's to the remarkable connection among people and Labradors — a bond based on adoration, trust, and faithful reliability. May your relationship with your Labrador be loaded up with vast undertakings, endless fondness, and a long period of esteemed recollections.

Wishing you and your Labrador
numerous cheerful years together,